Uma Geethanath

Tourettes Syndrome in Children and Young people: A Case series

Uma Geethanath

Tourettes Syndrome in Children and Young people: A Case series

Éditions universitaires européennes

Publisher:
Éditions universitaires européennes
is a trademark of
International Book Market Service Ltd., member of OmniScriptum Publishing Group
17 Meldrum Street, Beau Bassin 71504, Mauritius

Printed at: see last page
ISBN: 978-3-330-87082-6

Dedication

This book is dedicated to all the young people and their families I have seen in CYPS over the years.

 They have taught me most of what I know about Child Psychiatry, provide me with immense inspiration as well as sense of purpose and job satisfaction.

From them I have learnt an important message of acceptance, being appreciative and content with life in spite of the challenges it throws and learning to make the best of what you have.

I have also learnt how much of a difference it can make, having warm, understanding and supportive relationships around you.

I hope this case series will help other readers also to gain a better understanding of the above, in general and particularly in relation to Tourettes syndrome.

Table of Contents

Introduction

Tourette Syndrome (TS) is an inherited, neurological condition, characterised by multiple motor and vocal tics with onset before age 16 years.

Once thought to be a rare condition, the global prevalence is now estimated higher than previously thought, at about 1% (Robertson 2008) and is more common in males than females, about 3:1.

Tic symptoms have been reported since antiquity, but the condition was systematically studied and reported only from the 19th century by Itard (1825) and Gilles de la Tourette (1885).

It is a complex condition, covering a wide spectrum of symptoms, co-morbidities and severities. TS is often linked to other behaviours eg Obsessive Compulsive Disorder (OCD) and Attention Deficit Hyperactivity Disorder (ADHD). People with TS also often experience a range of associated symptoms such as anger, low mood which can sometimes be the most challenging aspects of the condition.

Overall this condition with its associated co-morbidities can lead to reduced quality of life for the young person, and high levels of stress for the parents and care givers. It could affect self esteem and self confidence as well as acceptance in family and social life, school and job performance.

There is no cure for TS, although different drugs and psychological therapies such as Cognitive Behavioural Therapy and Habit reversal training have been used successfully in a small number of TS patients.

None of these treatments completely eliminate symptoms and outcomes are variable depending on multiple factors.

Here we present a series of young people with Tourettes seen in a generic Tier 3 CAMHS clinic which demonstrates the complex interplay of the above issues. Having worked closely with these young people, each of them has helped me gain insight into a specific aspect of the condition, that I would like to share with my colleagues as well as other young people, parents and professionals working with this condition. Hopefully this will help us all to see beyond the Tics and get to know the young person underneath, and highlight areas of intervention that might make the biggest difference to their lives.

Key Observations

From observing our young people in this case series we noted that when the Tourettes Syndrome had been around for number of years, with symptom severity requiring trial of several different medications, over time, the medications seemed to prove less effective.

If reasonable symptom control was to be achieved, this tended to be within first few trials of medication. Understanding this at an early stage lead to acceptance and being able to adjust and move on.

Recognising and managing co-morbidities such as ADHD and low mood also seemed to be crucial.

Apart from symptom severity, other factors seemed to play a much bigger role in determining functioning ie having a warm accepting supportive family, supportive schooling environment, having another focus eg vocational college/ performing arts seemed to be associated with better functioning whereas psychosocial adversity, other challenging behavioural issues were associated with poor functioning.

High IQ with an excessive focus on the TS symptoms, was associated with more subjective distress, even when the symptoms were relatively mild.

Also high levels of parental anxiety, over protectiveness and excessive parental focus on the TS symptoms increased parental stress as well as increased reliance on medication.

Main learning points

In Tourettes Syndrome, the focus of assessments right from the beginning, needs to be on the associated psychosocial factors in addition to the symptoms themselves, as they seem to determine the functioning regardless of symptom severity.

Finding potential strengths and building on them, developing a focus on purposeful activities that can be handled despite ongoing TS symptoms, can lead to good functioning even with poor symptom control.

Also having a warm supportive family seems crucial to good functioning. Efforts need to be put in place to support the whole family so that they develop a shared understanding and acceptance of the TS and work together to manage it.

What are Tics, What is a Tic disorder, is Tourettes Syndrome different?

Tics

A Tic is a sudden repetitive movement, gesture or utterance.

They can occur in bouts with brief inter- Tic intervals.

They can occur singly or together in an orchestrated pattern. They vary in intensity and forcefulness.

Motor Tics vary from simple eye blinking, head jerking and shoulder shrugging to more complex facial expressions and hand gestures. In rare extreme cases they can be obscene gestures (copropraxia) or self-injurious (hitting or biting).

Phonic or vocal Tics can range from simple throat clearing to more complex utterances. In rare extreme cases coprolalia (obscene or socially unacceptable speech) is present.

Most individuals are aware of premonitory urges in a particular focal region or as a mental awareness when the Tic is about to occur (like an itch or a tickling sensation). Most patients also report a fleeting sense of relief after a bout of Tics. Most Tics can also be suppressed for brief periods of time.

Tic disorder

Transient Tic disorder:

This condition is diagnosed when a child has either one or more simple motor Tics that wax and wane in severity over weeks to months. There must be fewer than 12 consecutive months of active symptomatology. This is a retrospective diagnosis as it is difficult to predict at the outset which children will have self limiting symptoms and which will be progressive.

Chronic Motor Tic disorder:

This chronic condition is characterised by a waxing and waning course and broad range of severity of motor Tics, lasting more than 12 consecutive months and usually associated with other co-morbidities eg ADHD, however this isn't necessary.

Tourettes Syndrome:

This is the more severe combined motor and vocal Tic disorder. It typically starts with simple motor Tics around ages 2-4 yrs. The Tics come and go for a few years and progressively become more persistent.

The vocal Tics usually begin 1-2 years after the motor Tics.

The Tics characteristically wax and wane, are usually preceded by premonitory sensations, diminish during goal directed behaviour and increase with emotional excitement and fatigue.

The most common motor Tics begin in the head and neck areas, including eye blinking, eye rolling, pouting, grimacing, mouth stretching, head jerking etc and can get more complex eg touching, hopping, compulsive touching and sniffing.

Simple vocal Tics include sniffing, throat clearing, snorting, coughing, and complex Tics include spitting, barking, making animal noises, uttering strings of words.

Media often tend to include coprolalia (obscene or socially unacceptable speech) and copropraxia (obscene gestures) when portraying Tourettes syndrome, but this is quite rare ie only around 10% of severe Tourettes cases have this.

Other features include echolalia (copying what others say), palilalia (repeating the last part of ones sentences), echopraxia (copying what others do) and palipraxia (repeating one's own action).

The behavioural and emotional problems that frequently complicate TS range from impulsive, disinhibited and immature behaviours.

Although children with TS can be loving and affectionate, many find it particularly difficult to maintain age appropriate social skills. This could be because of the stigmatising effects of the Tics, the patient's own uneasiness but could also involve some fundamental neurodevelopmental difficulties linked to this condition.

Co-morbidity with Tourettes syndrome:
Both in clinic population and in the community, 90% have co-morbid Psychiatric conditions.

These include ADHD, ASD, Obsessive Compulsive behaviours, as well as internalising problems. They also are more likely to have anger control problems and sleep difficulties.

The subgroup of children with co-morbid ADHD are also more likely to have other associated disruptive behaviours such as aggression, delinquency and conduct problems, as well as poor social adaptation.

Obsessive Compulsive behaviours in people with TS include thoughts of violence, aggression and sex and compulsions involving touching of self and others, symmetry and ordering, rather than a fear of germs or contamination seen in OCD.

Other neurodevelopmental disorders:

Children with a range of developmental disorders are at increased risk for Tic disorders. These include Learning disabilities, specific learning difficulties, Speech impairments, physical impairments, Autism and pervasive developmental disorders.

Coexistent psychopathology:

Coexistent Depression and anxiety is common in TS. It might reflect the cumulative psychosocial burden of having Tics. The Depression severity is more closely associated with antecedent Psychosocial stress and obsessive compulsive symptoms than with measures of Tic severity.

Etiology:

Majority of Tourette's syndrome is inherited, although the exact mode of inheritance is not yet known and no gene has been identified.

There is a 50% chance of passing the gene to one of one's children.

But TS is a condition of variable expression and incomplete penetrance.
Males are more likely than females to express tics.

Autoimmune processes may affect tic onset and exacerbation in some cases, eg PANDAS (Paediatric autoimmune disorders associated with Streptococcal infection.

Some forms of obsessive compulsive behaviours may be genetically linked to Tourette's.

The precise mechanism of TS is unknown. Tics are believed to result from dysfunction in cortical and subcortical regions, the thalamus, basal ganglia and frontal cortex. Neuroanatomic models implicate failures in circuits connecting the brain's cortex and sub-cortex, and imaging techniques implicate the basal ganglia and frontal cortex.

Other causes of Tourettes like presentation/ Tourettism:
Some conditions might look like Tic disorders (Tic mimickers) eg Chorea, Myoclonus, Dystonia.

Some Genetic syndromes, some infectious/ post-infectious disorders and some Pervasive developmental disorders might have associated movement disorders that look loke like Tics.

Some patients might have Tics acquired from head injury, drugs and toxins.

Course of Tourettes Syndrome:
The peak severity of Tics is around ages 10-12 yrs, and plateau for a few years after this. The symptoms start improving by late adolescence and early adulthood, ie they decrease in severity.

A follow up study by Pappert et al (2003) showed that 90% of the adults followed up still had Tics. Even of those patients who reported being Tic free, more than 50% still had objective Tics. However only 13% of these adults were on medication, compared to 81% of the children. The authors concluded that Tics improve with time but most adults still have Tics.

Another study by Rizzo et al (2012) showed that at follow up, people with pure Tourettes syndrome (no co-morbidity) in childhood had a better prognosis and better quality of life, and less need for medication compared to the people with co-morbid conditions from childhood.

However some of the most severe and debilitating forms of Tic disorder can also be found in adulthood. The factors that influence continuity of symptoms from childhood to adolescence to adulthood are not fully understood. They might involve the interplay between normal maturational processes, exposure to drugs such as Cocaine, stimulants and steroids, the amount of intramorbid emotional trauma and distress, Psychological stress, activation of immune system etc.

The factors that determine the degree of disability and handicap versus resilience is unknown.

They are likely to include the presence of additional developmental disorders, level of support and understanding from parents, teachers and peers, the presence of special abilities (eg sport or performing arts) or personal attributes (intelligence, social abilities and personality traits).

Treatment options:
There is no cure for Tourette's and no medication that works universally for all individuals.

Tourette's treatment mainly focuses on Psychoeducation, and Cognitive and Behavioural techniques to help the individual manage the most troubling or impairing symptoms, and providing peer support.

Medication can be useful for symptomatic relief:

Clonidine (alpha 2 agonist) is generally tried first when medication is needed, due to less side effects. Antipsychotics ie Haloperidol, Pimozide, Risperidone etc have some proven efficacy to reduce the intensity of the Tics, atleast in the short term. Stimulants or Atomoxetine are used for co-morbid ADHD. SSRIs are used for co-morbid OCD and Depression.

Newer treatments, still not mainstream, may be available to adults: Botox injection, Medical Cannabis (not in U.K.), Deep brain stimulation.

Support groups eg Support organisations like Tourettes Action are most helpful in providing patients and their families with a better understanding of the condition, promoting acceptance and providing much needed hope and optimism as well as giving practical advice about accessing other support in the community. They also provide information and support to professionals working with TS and fund much needed research in this area.

Behavioural treatments:

Behavioural therapy can be useful for most people with tic disorders, it is more effective for children older than 8 yrs and adults.

The most commonly validated behavioural therapy is Habit Reversal Therapy (HRT). HRT is more effective as part of a package alongside other elements of therapy, this is known as Comprehensive Behavioural Intervention for Tics (CBiT).

CBiT is a combination of the following elements:

- Psychoeducation;
- Relaxation techniques;

- CBT for co-morbid anxiety and OCD, etc.;
- Functional Analysis;
- Habit reversal Training;
- Exposure and Response prevention.

Functional analysis:

Functional analysis is used to identify environmental events that make tics worse or maintain tics for an individual. A therapist will help a person with tics to understand what tends to happen before and after a bout of tics.

This may include reactions to situation, thoughts or feelings that a person has in a particular place and the way in which other people respond to that person when they tic.

The therapist will then work with the person to reduce or get rid of tic increasing situations. Relaxation or the ability to look at the situation in another way may help.

Habit Reversal training:

This is geared towards control of individual Tics.

The **first stage of HRT is tic description and awareness**.

Increasing the persons' sense of when a tic is about to happen, called a premonitory urge will help them to control it.

The **next stage is picking the most problematic Tic and finding a competing response**. This trains the person to perform an intentional movement, which means that the tic cannot happen. Eg for a Tic involving flinging their arm out, they can be taught to channel the premonitory urge into something more favourable such as placing their hand on their leg and pushing gently. People can get really good at creating their own competing responses once they understand the principle of how to do it.

Exposure and Response prevention ie Habituation:

Theoretically there is fluctuation of premonitory urges in TS, both naturally and during ERP:

1) In natural fluctuation: urge rises- tic happens- urge decreases
2) In ERP: urge rises – tics are prevented – urge reaches a top and decrease without giving in to a tic.

The more the person trains this, (s) he will habituate to this process and the top of the sensation-curve will decrease. Eventually the person can endure the sensation without continuously manifesting tics.

Cases 1 and 2

Supportive accepting family, pleasant temperament, fighting attitude to life even with severe Tourettes syndrome

These 2 young men, identical twins, were among the first most severe cases of TS that I had met since starting as a Consultant Child and Adolescent Psychiatrist 9 years ago.

At the time they were 10 yrs old and had already been seeing my senior colleague Consultant for 2-3 yrs.

If they were in the waiting area the whole department was aware as they had quite explosive vocal Tics and motor Tics and tended to bounce off each other.

One of the twins had more significant learning difficulties than the other, both boys also had co-morbid ADHD.

By the time I got to took over their care the boys had already been tried on 3 different antipsychotics, and had already been seen for second opinion in the local paediatric neurology clinic as well as the Tourettes clinic in Great Ormond Street Hospital.
However when I met the boys and started getting to know them well, what stood out most was their very pleasant personalities.

They were both always smiling, chatty and maintained their positivity inspite of how severe the Tics were.

They had a good sense of humour. They also had a lot of self confidence, were secure in their peer relationships, well liked and accepted by their teachers and peers. They were very determined lads and kept pushing themselves and carried on functioning ie attending school and extracurricular activities no matter what.

Both boys received an Education Healthcare Plan and were placed in a Special school for Emotional and Behavioural difficulties when they moved to secondary school. Therefore they were taught in small classes with high level of staffing and a more practical curriculum and scope to use a more flexible and tailored approach to education.

What also stood out throughout was the warmth and acceptance within the family and the commitment of both parents. The parents were totally in tune with the boys, they had endless patience and time for them. Even though like most parents they were always trying and hoping to find that medication or that dose change that might relieve the boys of some of the intensity of their Tics, they accepted the boys fully as they were. They were always gentle with the boys and seemed to be able to maintain a calm soothing effect on them. It wasn't always easy and the family had their own share of other psychosocial stresses. There were times when parents felt quite worn out themselves but this did not get projected on to the boys.

Throughout the 7-8 years that I have been working with the boys, the severity of their Tics waxed and waned but they were never symptom free. There were periods when it was really intense with explosive shouting out spitting, jumping on the spot, hitting oneself on the face and abdomen etc.

Behavioural therapies were tried but the boys found it difficult to take these techniques on board and put into action.

They had gone a full circle with various antipsychotics and Clonidine for the TS and various medication for the ADHD. We still kept trying, going back to medication that had been benefitial in the past hoping that they might work again after a break.

It was difficult to know if any of the symptoms reductions were due to medication changes or if it was the natural course of waxing and waning but it seemed to give the family the satisfaction that we were trying.

Support groups such as the Tourettes Action were mentioned to the family on numerous occassions but they did not feel the need to access these.
Instead the boys attended local youth clubs and activities available through the Disabilities team.

Both boys managed to go through school without getting into the wrong crowd, without getting into any complications like substance misuse or delinquent behaviours.

After leaving school one of the twins joined an animal care course at College and is adjusting really well, enjoying the course. The other twin has joined an apprenticeship in a kitchen with a catering company. He is also coping vey well with his job. They are both happy and content with themselves.

Both boys now 19 yrs, still have significant Tics, are still on medication for the ADHD and the TS, and have been transferred to adult Neurology clinic to look at other treatment options.

Case 3

Impact of temperament, co-morbidities, psychosocial stresses, and lack of appropriate support

This young man I have been seeing since he was 9 yrs. He has helped me understand the course of severe Tourettes as well as the impact of various complicating factors on the direction this condition can take.

When I first starting seeing him, he has already had simple motor and vocal Tics for a couple of years. He also had associated low frustration tolerance and emotional regulation issues for which he was receiving some therapeutic input from a school counsellor and referred to our service for these symptoms.

He was otherwise a lively young man, bright, sporty, well liked by teachers and popular amongst his peers, inspite of being a bit strong willed.

When seen in clinic, he presented as a pleasant young man, but had difficulty sustaining focus in the sessions, low frustration tolerance, and so did his mom. They would often have several things going on at once, get stressed easily and often cancelled appointments. At that stage mom was keen for something to fix him and would often compare him with his younger brother who was neurotypical, hoping the same for him.

We tried to offer talking therapies with our Psychologists, both to the young man and also family sessions with him and mom to help them with Psychoeducation and accepting the condition, but by this time the Tics were getting more intense and it was understandably difficult for them.

They had practical support in the form of a Support worker from the Childrens services helping mom with de-escalation techniques, and helping the lad with emotional regulation as the high expressed emotions in the household was a big issue.

By the next 2 years, our young man was constantly having facial Tics, hand jerks, leg jerks, could not even walk in a straight line, was shouting out a lot.
Various antipsychotic medications were tried and each had some benefit for few months and then the next bout of Tics were more intense and they were no longer effective.

School was understanding and flexible while he was still in primary education, and still promoted his strengths in sports that kept his self-esteem and self-confidence up.

However he did not receive the Education and Healthcare plan inspite of our recommendations and moved to a mainstream secondary school. They did their best to support him but it was too much for him to handle, his explosive anger outbursts became a major issue alongside his complex Tics.
He lost most of his friends through this, could no longer keep up with his competitive sports and also fell behind academically. This had a negative impact on his mood.

Also by this time mom wasn't coping with it all and looked to his estranged dad to support him during times of crises. He got caught between the two parents who did not get along and were very critical of each other, blamed each other for his condition.

Then the family moved to a different area for mom's work reasons, it took several months for our lad to get into a local school. He drifted into the wrong crowd, started drinking alcohol and smoking Cannabis, stealing to fund his habit, got into physical fight with young people in the neighbourhood and received a community order for this.

Initially the Cannabis seemed to calm the Tics when they had stopped responding to our medication. So our lad decided this was his solution and started smoking it more and more on a daily basis. He lost all motivation in his studies, sports, friendships, disengaged from everything, continued to have explosive temper outbursts at home and in school. By now he was in a special school for emotional and behavioural difficulties, but did not cope there either and ended up not going or getting excluded.

Both mom and dad could not handle his behaviours and he was placed in Voluntary residential care.

He was once again well liked by staff but continued to use Cannabis a lot, became increasingly challenging and defiant, did not engage in any productive activities on offer. He would sleep most of the day and only get up to go out for his Cannabis, and even started bringing it in to the home. He developed drug induced psychosis needing a Psychiatric admission for a few weeks.

Since then he has been in 3 care homes as the homes could not tolerate the extent of his drug use and lack of engagement. He left school with no qualifications. Both parents are reluctant to have him with them, even for contacts, as they have other children in the house and worry about the impact of his behaviours and drug use on them.

He tried getting a job but his mind was so preoccupied and craving for drugs all the time that he could not hold it down. However he still finds it difficult to commit to the Community drug and alcohol service and engage in therapies to help him overcome the habit. He requested Psychiatric admission to help him break the vicious cycle but wasn't accepted as community options hadn't been tried first.

He is now nearly 18 yrs and his situation remains the same in terms of drug use and poor functioning. The tics are barely visible now, not the factor impacting on his functioning at all, even though he is only on a very small dose of antipsychotic medication.

Case 4

Role of support organisations, need for adequate Educational support, importance of having a sound hobby

This boy has helped me understand yet another aspect of Tourettes ie the role of good peer support organisations.

He has been seen in my clinics since age 11-12 yrs and has just been discharged aged 18 yrs.

Alongside his TS he also has Autism Spectrum disorder and specific learning difficulties (Dyslexia). Over the last 2 years he has also developed recurrent Depression.

He is a very pleasant, likeable and friendly young man. He is mild natured, keeps positive, is always willing to try strategies offered to him, has a "give it a go" attitude. He also keeps trying, doesn't give up hope easily. His mom is very understanding and supportive, accepts him as he is and tries her best to help him in any way she can, to achieve his goals.

His main Tics from the beginning have been his head bobbing, it can go on and on at times all day. In the recent years he has also been having complex vocal Tics where he shouts out inappropriate things or has very loud startling barking Tic.

When he first started secondary school aged 11 yrs, the Tics were not as bad, but he was bullied by peers due to his innocent nature, called "thick", was regularly provoked for a reaction. He also found the pace of the academic work too difficult to keep up with. The teachers did not really understand his social and emotional vulnerability and could not support him adequately in that setting. He missed a lot of education, kept getting sent home as Tics were too bad, had to be on part time table in a room by himself and did not really cope with it all.

After a lot of time and effort he finally got his Education Healthcare and was placed in another school with an ASD provision.

Here he had access to higher staffing levels, teaching in small groups, tailored curriculum. He had a more sympathetic peer group, started growing in self confidence and social skills also improved. He had access to a quiet sensory room he could use when Tics were too bad, but he could still stay on in school. He also was able to showcase his talent in music, drumming, he joined the school band and gave various performances, this improved his self confidence a lot. He also recognised that when he was fully focused on drumming a complex rhythm, keeping to the exact counts in his head, the head bobbing Tic calmed down for a bit.

By this time our lad had accessed Habit reversal training and other behavioural techniques to manage his Tics. He got the gist of it and was able to identify his own strategies. He also accepted that the strategies would not always work and on a bad day he just had to take it easy and let the Tics take its time to pass.

He had been tried on Clonidine and various antipsychotics and had also been seen in the second opinion clinic in Great Ormond Street Hospital. He and mom understood the limits of what medication could achieve and used it as a back up when things got too intense, to take the edge off rather than hoping to cure the Tics.

Our young man and his mom also engaged very well with support organisations like Tourettes action, joined their social groups, attended their Residential activities. He got to know a few older people with the condition who acted as his guides and mentors. Seeing them achieve in life inspite of their conditions gave him the hope that he could too. He learnt to accept his condition better and so did mom.

They also got a lot of useful practical ideas about how to cope while in public when the Tics were really bad and everybody was noticing. He learnt to have set things to say, even got himself a jumper with a brief message explaining it is just his Tourettes.

His Tics are still just as intense. He has also developed recurrent Depression over the last 2 years, and this is getting in the way of his functioning more than his TS. When low he is really tired, finds it difficult to get out of bed and face the world. But he doesn't let it take over, tries to maintain a basic routine as far as possible, and with medication and support and encouragement from mom, manages to get out of it.

He has finished school now and is attending College courses, trying various options to find himself a vocation. He says he really wants to get some GCSEs, train to be a special needs teacher and wants to inspire other young people that like him, wants to show them that they can also overcome their difficulties and achieve if they put their mind to it.

Case 5

Play to your strengths

This is another young man who will always remain fresh in my mind. I had been seeing him for a few years from ages 11 to 14 yrs but since then he has moved to America for his career reasons.

The thing I remember most about him is how good he was as an entertainer. He had an excellent sense of humour, was very good at pulling magic tricks, delivering jokes. In his reviews he preferred to get the necessary things out of the way as soon as possible and then try and impress me with his tricks. He was also very good at singing and drama. Mom had informed me that while on stage performing, there was no sign of his Tics.

This lad had started having Tics from the age of about 7-8 yrs, it had been triggered following him being assaulted in the face. It had started as simple facial Tics that waxed and waned but over the next few years, it increased to more persistent and more complex motor and vocal Tics.

He was also very fidgety, excitable, found it difficult sit still and concentrate in lessons, was impulsive, shouting out, getting into trouble. He ended up receiving an additional diagnosis of ADHD.

He was an only child and mom was very protective, worried a lot about him and his Tics and also about giving him any treatments and the potential side effects. He was on small doses of stimulant medication for his ADHD and on antipsychotics on and off for his Tics. He had therapeutic sessions with a nurse to help him with his emotional regulation issues.

The Tics increased in intensity through secondary school. They did not seem to bother him as much but seeing him Tic in this way was more of a struggle for mom.

However he got a major break a couple of years back, in a TV company in America doing teen music and soaps, advertisements etc. He started spending several months a year in America doing his projects, was well looked after there, had 1:1 private education arranged for him. He would be back in school in U.K. only briefly in between projects, mainly to catch up with friends. I was informed that this arrangement suited him really well. He was able to keep the Tics in check while at work and then could Tic as much as he needed to outside of this time.
He chose not to take his medication as it dampened his personality, and the Tics were not interfering with his functioning anyway.

Case 6

Importance of having another focus and also remember to address co-morbidities

This is a young lady with Tics I have been seeing from age 9-10 yrs, she is now 15 years.

She has various facial Tics including eye blinking, mouth stretching, picking at her skin and vocal tics including throat clearing, that waxed and waned.

She also has specific learning difficulties ie Dyscalculia, anxiety and emotional regulation issues, social insecurity and social relatedness issues.

When first seen she wasn't even aware of her Tics and it was these emotional regulation issues, social insecurity and social relatedness issues that caused her the most problems in school.

Both her parents were on the teaching profession, the worked closely with the school, ensured she had Psychometric assessment and necessary support and differentiation for her Dyscalculia.

As she matured and moved to secondary school, she was better able to manage her emotional regulation issues in school compared to primary school. Parents arranged a tight transition plan between primary and secondary school and had regular meetings. She coped with the increased academic demands of secondary school better than expected. If there were any hiccups parents were able to liaise with school and get them resolved straight away. She improved her social skills and social confidence, although it wasn't always easy for her.

Parents encouraged her and tried to find her opportunities to refine her social skills and improve her self confidence. She was in a drama group and attended practice every weekend and also performed in shows. However as she grew older she started getting tired of this.

Over the last couple of years she has joined a rowing club and has been attending several times a week. She has recognised a special talent there and started entering competitions and doing really well. This has given her a big boost to her confidence.

Also, in the rowing club she has found a group of like minded friends with similar interests. She sees them socially, has been going out with them, has sleep overs. She feels totally at ease with them and this has improved her social confidence a lot.

There were times when things got too much, she got overwhelmed, anxious, her mood dipped. She even suffered from an episode of Depression. But her parents were tuned in to her needs, were very supportive throughout.

The Tics still come and go but not have a significant impact on her functioning. She is only takes antipsychotic medication for it when it gets too intense, to take the edge off. She is on regular anxiolytic medication though.

Having the structure and regular routine of the rowing club has helped her keep going when things got tough, helped her cope with her emotional regulation issues and even helped her overcome her Depression.

Case 7

Could be another underlying organic cause

This young girl is 9 yrs old. I have only seen a couple of times in clinic myself, and was previously seen by our Senior Registrar a year ago.

She had quite typical presentation of motor and vocal Tics as well as obsessive compulsive behaviours, for 2-3 years.

She also has associated episodic increased emotionality and heightened separation anxiety symptoms.

She presentsed in clinic as a very calm, sensible mature child for her age. She was generally very well behaved at home and school, doing well academically and socially. There were some Psychosocial factors in the background and she was quite tuned in to the impact of these on her parents, looking out for them.

Alongside the waxing and waning Tics she also had episodic increase in her emotionality and separation anxiety, not necessarily associated with throat infections. Mom had read up about PANDAS (Paediatric autoimmune neuropsychiatric disorders associated with streptococcal infections) and suspected this in her child. She sought referrals and was seen by neurologist who suggested chorea and immunologist who suggested PANDAS.

She has been on prophylactic antibiotics and now awaiting Tonsillectomy, due to the possible link with PANDAS. She has also had trials of various antipsychotic medication before this with limited success.

At present the Tics do not seem to have too much of an impact on her functioning and the girl is not particularly distressed by them. Mom however is understandably anxious seeing her daughter having so many Tics and is keen to find a cure for her condition.

Mom also accepts the emotional impact of her other Psychosocial factors, sees this as a separate issue and is willing for her to have some therapeutic support around this, she is awaiting allocation for this.

Case 8

Parental anxiety can be a significant factor that needs to be picked up and addressed

This very pleasant young man is 12 years old and has been having vocal and motor Tics for last 3-4 years.

It was initially present on and off, but has been present more or less continuously for the last 1 ½ years. This includes mainly head jerking, facial tics and throat clearing and nowadays he has them throughout the day.

Our lad is otherwise very calm and settled, does well academically and is well adjusted socially, he has no behavioural issues at home or school other than the Tics.

He reports some discomfort when he has been having the Tics all day, sometimes it gets very distracting and he cannot concentrate in lessons.
However he manages to catch up, his peers and teachers are understanding and supportive.

The family have had Psychoeducation, have been offered details regarding Tourettes action support groups. But mom is still at the stage where she is looking for a cure.

Mom feels very distressed seeing her child having the Tics all day, is keen for him to have medication to contain the Tics. He has had trials of Clonidine and four different antipsychotics and an SSRI. He did not respond well enough to any of these and had side effects, needing them to be changed. But mom is still on the look out for other medications, worrying constantly and contacting the service every week to see if medication dose can be increased further.

He has been seen in the second opinion paediatric neuropsychiatry clinic but feels a bit disappointed that no new medication has been suggested as yet.

Cases 9 and 10

I have Tics, so what?

These boys, both aged 10 years have only been seen in the service on and off.

They have both had vocal and motor Tics since age 4 yrs. They used to come and go but for the last year they have been around most of the time.

Also previously they were able to subconsciously keep it under control in school but in the last year it has been more noticeable in school, peers have started questioning them.

However apart from these Tics these boys are neurotypical, have no academic, social or behavioural issues. They are confident, outgoing, and popular with friends.

They are both not distressed by the Tics are generally able to get on with it.

Both sets of parents have had psychoeducation, done their own research on the subject and are well informed about TS. They are very understanding and supportive.

They have spoken with school teachers about the condition so they can be more accommodating and be able to address it with peers if there is any teasing.

They had only come to the service for reassurance and advice regarding whether they need to be doing anything more for their children to prevent further escalation of the Tics.

They were able to take on board information about the probable course of the condition and various treatment options available in future but for now to let them get on with their lives when they are coping so well.

Both sets of parents agreed that their children were coping with the condition better than they were , they felt need to have support in coming to terms with it and plan to access support groups like Tourettes Action.

Final words about Tourettes Syndrome

Tourettes has no cure. Treatments at best help one to manage the condition rather than eliminate it.

Co-morbidity is common in TS and they come in a wide range of complexity and intensity. Also the associated psychosocial factors seem to determine the functioning regardless of symptom severity.

A supportive environment and family generally gives those with Tourette's the skills and ability to function and to manage the disorder better.

Even outcomes in adulthood are associated more with the perceived significance of having severe tics as a child than with the actual severity of the tics.

The main focus of intervention needs to be gaining a full understanding of the individual, their strengths and difficulties, co-morbidities, and try and maximise acceptance and positive regard irrespective of the Tics.

It is most helpful to see the TS as only an aspect of the person and identify the whole person underneath the Tics, help them identify their unique strengths and talents and make the best of these.

The more others are aware of the condition eg parents, School, College, work place etc, the better for the person's self confidence and self esteem, and the easier it will be for them to make the necessary adjustment to allow the young person to achieve their full potential.

There may be latent advantages associated with an individual's genetic vulnerability to developing Tourette, eg. a heightened awareness and increased attention to detail and surroundings, that may have adaptive value.

People with Tourette's may learn to camouflage or to channel the energy of their tics into a functional endeavour.

Accomplished musicians, athletes, public speakers and professionals from all walks of life are found among people with Tourette's. Having adequate support and contact with other people with TS is important in providing hope and positive role models to look up to.

References

1. Tourettes Syndrome in Children and Adolescents: aetiology, presentation and treatment, BJPsych Advances (2016), vol 22, pg 165-175.

2. Danielle C. Cath, Jeremy Stern, Tara Murphy et al, European clinical guidelines for Tourette Syndrome and other tic disorders, Part I: assessment, Eur Child Adolesc Psychiatry. 2011 Apr; 20(4): 155--171.

3. Daniel A. Gorman, Nancy Thompson, Kerstin J. Plessen, Mary M. Robertson, James F. Leckman and Bradley S. Peterson, Psychosocial outcome and psychiatric comorbidity in older adolescents with Tourette syndrome: controlled study, BJP 2010, 197:36-44.

4. Carter AS, O'Donnell DA, Schultz RT, Scahill L, Leckman JF, Pauls DL. Social and emotional adjustment in children affected with Gilles de la Tourette's syndrome: associations with ADHD and family functioning. J Child Psychol Psychiatry 2000; 41: 215–23.